EAT MORE, DO LESS, GET FIT

EAT MORE, DO LESS, GET FIT

Health and Fitness for Everyone

A simple and easy to follow guide that anyone can use to achieve their health and fitness goals

DAN COLLINS
ISAA Certified Personal Trainer and Nutritionist

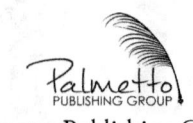

Palmetto Publishing Group
Charleston, SC

Eat More, Do Less, Get Fit
Copyright © 2020 by Dan Collins

All rights reserved

All rights reserved. This book or any portion thereof may not be reproduced or used in any manner whatsoever without the express written permission of the publisher except for the use of brief quotations in a book review.

First Edition

Printed in the United States

ISBN-13: 978-1-64111-783-8
ISBN-10: 1-64111-783-4

Disclaimer: This is not medical advice. Please consult your doctor before beginning this or any fitness and nutrition program.

TABLE OF CONTENTS

Foreword · vii
Introduction ·ix
Chapter 1   Nutrition · 1
Chapter 2   Training · 16
Chapter 3   My Story · 26
Chapter 4   Living the Eat More, Do Less, Get Fit Lifestyle · · · · · · · · 30
Chapter 5   Supplements · 34

FOREWORD
Written by my dear friend Jeff Brown

The ketogenic (keto) diet and similar diets that have been around for a long time, like the Atkins diet and its progeny, are all over the news now: "Want a Better Night's Sleep? The Keto Diet Can Help"[1] or "Keto Diet Stops Growth of Certain Cancers, Study Suggests."[2] Or how about "Ketogenic Diets as an Adjuvant Cancer Therapy: History and Potential Mechanism"?[3] These headlines, and the various ways to get on keto or stay on keto, are a sign of the times: Americans are generally out of shape and overweight. More than one in three Americans is medically "obese." That means more than just a few pounds "overweight." It means your body mass index, or BMI, is bigger than thirty. That's the measure that medical professionals use to determine your fatness, calculated with a specific mathematical formula,[4] comparing your height to your weight. And the average person who is one or both of those things—out of shape and/or overweight—wants to do something about it but doesn't know where to start, what to do, or who to believe.

I've known Dan Collins for over forty years. I've worked with and for him as a counselor, advisor, attorney, and friend. (Also as a housepainter

---

1 Stephanie Booth, "Want a Better Night's Sleep? The Keto Diet Can Help," Healthline, January 24, 2019, https://www.healthline.com/health-news/keto-diet-improves-sleep.
2 Bailey King, "Keto Diet Stops Growth of Certain Cancers, Study Suggests," *Philly Voice*, August 14, 2019, https://www.phillyvoice.com/ketogenic-diet-stops-cancer-tumor-growth-study/.
3 Bryan G. Allen, "Ketogenic Diets as an Adjuvant Cancer Therapy: History and Potential Mechanism," *Redox Biology* 2 (2014): 963-970, https://www.ncbi.nlm.nih.gov/pmc/articles/PMC4215472/.
4 BMI is calculated as (weight in pounds x 703) ÷ (height in inches).

and a retail clerk when we were in high school together.) Ever since I can remember, Dan was interested in physical health, wellness, and fitness. As Dan freely admits in this book, Dan was once the stereotypical scrawny teenager at the beach, but the difference between him and most others was that he decided to do something about it. And then he did it. In a remarkably short period of time in his late teens, Dan went from scrawny to substantial, sizeable, and sturdy.

Unlike a lot of people I've known, however, Dan has managed to stay fit and healthy over the past forty years. Most people who meet Dan for the first time guess that he is five to ten years younger (or more) than he really is. I've seen those introductions and surprise "reveals" with reactions of genuine disbelief, time and again. And that's been increasingly true as we've gotten older.

But there's really no magic here. This is simply Dan doing what his book is saying, walking the walk while talking the talk. The goals set forth in his book are very attainable for the average person. The steps to be taken are most definitely incremental—you don't read the book, then walk to the mirror and observe transformation on the spot. Instead, Dan gives you all the basic information, written in a straightforward and understandable manner, that you need in order to transform yourself. Then it is up to you. It is always up to you.

If you are interested in a permanent, healthful change, then you owe it to yourself to read this book and follow its advice. I wish and hope for you the best. You must do the rest.

Eat More, Do Less, Get Fit

INTRODUCTION

In today's world it seems like everything has to be taken to the *extreme*. This is especially true in the world of fitness. *Extreme* diets. *Extreme* workouts. *Extreme* results. Well, I am here to tell you that you can accomplish everything you want without having to go to the *extreme*. Eat More, Do Less, Get Fit is based on the simple idea of combining a healthy, macronutrient-balanced nutrition plan with an appropriate and effective workout routine to *Eat More, Do Less, Get Fit!*

My goal is to explain the Eat More, Do Less, Get Fit concept using everyday terms and anecdotal examples from my own life to illustrate the concept and provide a foundation for you to do the same. I started my fitness journey long ago when I was just a teenager. Unfortunately, the commonly accepted fitness theory at the time was *"More is better"*—the complete opposite of what I discovered to be true and have now compiled into the Eat More, Do Less, Get Fit vision.

I was the quintessential ninety-pound weakling in my teens. That is when I decided to *"Get huge"*. I joined a gym, started lifting weights, and also tried to eat everything in sight, by what was known back then as the *"See Food Diet"*—if I saw it, I'd try to eat it! The *"More is better"* theory applied to nutrition in the same way it applied to training, and it was so far off the mark. Eat More, Do Less, Get Fit explains the error within this practice and the importance of a macronutrient-balanced approach to nutrition planning. *Eat More!*

Back then everything, and I do mean everything, was *"More is better"*. This was applied to any sort of diet plan, workout routine, anything and everything related to fitness. I believe this is where the *extreme* workout routines began as well. Unfortunately, this is also as far from the truth as you could possibly get. *Do Less!*

I hope you are as excited about the prospects of an effective yet reasonable health and fitness plan that you can actually do without going to the *extreme*. By combining a sound nutritional plan along with an appropriate training program, you can achieve your personal health and fitness goals. Eat More, Do Less, Get Fit is exactly that. *Get Fit!*

CHAPTER 1:
NUTRITION

Eat More, Do Less, Get Fit will show that the current common thoughts about diet and fitness are simply incorrect. First let's talk diet, or rather nutrition. Then we can add in the training routine which I am sure will surprise you just as much as what I am now going to tell you about nutrition!

Nutrition planning is critical to a successful health and fitness plan. It is the very foundation on which fitness is built, and this statement sums it all up.

> **Whatever you achieve in the gym will be revealed by what is on your plate.**

Diet is typically where most popular fitness plans fail right out of the gate. Most diets rely on a restrictive list of approved foods that do not satisfy your hunger and leave you feeling empty and miserable. Couple that with maniacal workouts like what you see in Peloton commercials or the one-size-fits-all workouts that the personal trainers at most big chain gyms offer, and all you have is a recipe for quitting—and who could blame you?

Instead of diet, I prefer to use the term "nutrition planning." This is a much more palatable approach where you look at what you are eating and decide how quickly you want to reach the goals you have set for yourself. Then you simply eat your way there.

The biggest mistake I see in most nutrition plans is a misunderstanding of macronutrients, especially when it comes to simple and processed carbohydrates. There is a mistaken belief that eating fat makes you fat. This is so far from the truth. The truth is that eating high-glycemic, simple, processed carbohydrates that cause *extreme* sugar spikes and crashes is what actually creates body fat. Eating based on a nutrition plan that focuses on balancing the macronutrients that you consume is the key to burning fat—not hours in the gym sweating up a storm, doing endless cardio workouts. Remember—everything you create in the gym will be revealed by what's on your plate.

So, what are macronutrients? These are the basic compounds that are identified on every nutrition label: carbohydrates, proteins, and fats. These nutrients are what food is comprised of, but depending on the specific food, they are distributed in different ratios. For instance, fruits and grains are comprised largely of simple carbohydrates or, more accurately, sugar. Proteins are comprised of amino acids, which are the building blocks of all tissue within your body, especially muscle. And fats are compounds that your body uses to perform various internal functions such as hormone production and maintenance. Each macronutrient serves a very specific function within your body, and the secret to Eat More, Do Less, Get Fit is to eat these macronutrients in the right ratios. By eating them in the correct ratios, you can create the physique that you want. Whether that is to reduce fat and sculpt your body into a lean physique or to build muscle and gain weight. Whatever your goal, you can accomplish it through the Eat More, Do Less, Get Fit program.

Let's get started by discussing carbohydrates and their role in the body. Carbohydrates, unlike fats, are what actually make you fat. Yes. You read that correctly. Carbohydrates, unlike fats, are what actually make you fat. It is the roller coaster ride of blood sugar spikes and crashes caused by consuming simple, processed carbohydrates that causes your body to build and retain fat tissue, and here's why. As you consume simple carbohydrates, your blood sugar spikes and crashes, which your body interprets as an emergency situation that it needs to compensate for by creating and utilizing body fat.

BLOOD SUGAR SPIKES & CRASHES

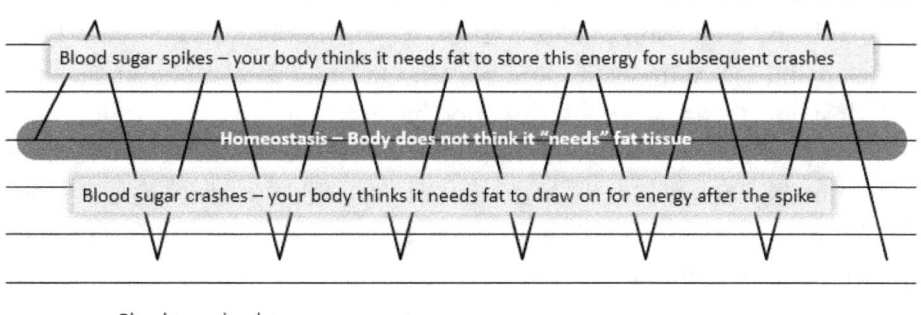

Simple, processed carbohydrates are high-glycemic-index foods. What is the glycemic index? The glycemic index is a scale that you can use to determine how fast your body will convert carbohydrates into glucose. The speed at which a carbohydrate is converted into glucose will directly affect how fast and how much your blood sugar level will spike. This is important because two foods with the exact same number of carbohydrates but with different glycemic index values will affect your blood sugar in very different ways.

The glycemic index ranges from zero to one hundred, and white table sugar is about a seventy on the index, which is considered quite high. Wheat flour and high-fructose corn syrup, which are used in practically every processed food in the world, have extremely high glycemic index values too! What this means is that when you consume these types of simple, processed carbohydrate-rich foods, your blood sugar jumps almost immediately and uncontrollably. This is especially true when you consume white table sugar. Science has shown that white table sugar can actually enter your bloodstream directly through the tissues in your mouth, throat, and stomach without any sort of governing mechanism. This unregulated entry of simple sugars into your blood supply gives you that sudden burst of energy but then, once exhausted, is quickly followed by a subsequent drop in blood sugar, which leaves you sluggish and empty. This tells your body that it now needs to compensate by accessing fat stores for energy or, worse yet, you may just consume more simple, processed carbohydrates triggering yet another blood sugar spike and crash! This can become a vicious cycle of blood sugar spikes and crashes that further encourages your body to create and maintain even more body fat in order to compensate.

Most meat and vegetables do not have a high glycemic index. Red meat, eggs, chicken, cheese, and nuts all have a glycemic index of zero since they contain very few carbohydrates. These high fat and protein foods also have to be processed through the liver, which regulates how fast they are released into the blood supply. Vegetables such as asparagus, brussel sprouts, kale, and broccoli all have a very low glycemic index of less than twenty because they have some carbohydrates but also fiber, which reduces their net carbohydrates. I will explain net carbohydrates a little later on. So you can see why it is much more advantageous to eat meat and vegetables rather than simple, processed carbohydrates or large amounts of fruit and fruit juice, which are also high on the glycemic index when compared to foods high in fats, proteins, and fiber.

Your body works best in a state of *"homeostasis"*. Homeostasis is basically a fancy term for a consistent blood sugar level. Whenever your body is out of homeostasis, it will believe that it *"needs"* fat, and here is why. When your blood sugar spikes, your body will believe that it needs fat to store this excess energy in order to compensate for the subsequent blood sugar level crashes. When your blood sugar level crashes, your body will again believe it needs the fat to supply energy to compensate for the crash. Both situations tell your body it needs fat! Fats and proteins do not create this sort of spike and crash within your body. They are digested and processed through your liver, which governs how fast they are released into your blood supply as illustrated in the following chart.

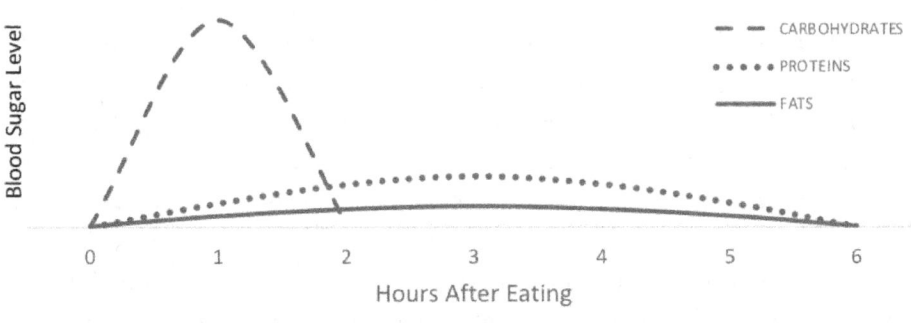

How Macronutrients Affect Blood Sugar Levels

Here is where the other shoe drops when it comes to the belief that *extreme* cardio can address this issue by creating a calorie deficit and thereby burning body fat. This, again, is an erroneous assumption that I see many people making in the gym. I am not saying cardio is not beneficial. It is, but only when you work out within your fat-burning target heart rate zone. Working out above or below your fat-burning target heart rate zone will not burn fat in any meaningful way even though it may create an overall calorie deficiency.

Cardio work above your target heart rate zone will only burn readily available energy already in your cells. Once this supply is exhausted, which happens within a matter of minutes, your body will turn to lean tissue to create energy because this process is simpler and quicker than converting body fat to energy. On top of this, because your body still believes it needs fat stores to compensate for blood sugar spikes and crashes, it will not burn body fat since it believes it is necessary to help maintain a state of homeostasis. Instead it will turn to lean tissue for energy.

Along with this, now you have created a situation where your body has exhausted its quick energy supply, and once you finish the workout, your body will crave even more high-glycemic carbohydrates, which most people will consume. This defeats the very idea that your body will be forced to burn fat because of your *extreme* cardio workout. We will circle back to this later when we start talking about fitness training.

Proteins and fats, on the other hand, are digested and then processed through your liver, where they are turned into amino acids and fatty acids that are used to rebuild tissue, create other proteins, and even used to produce energy when you follow a balanced macronutrient nutrition plan. Proteins and fats do not cause blood sugar spikes, nor do they make you fat—unless you consume them as part of a diet that is far in excess of your daily requirements. This is not where we need to focus other than to explain where proteins and fats can be found.

Proteins can be found in both animal and plant sources. The key difference between the two is the *"completeness"* of the protein. A complete protein is one that contains all twenty amino acids.

There is a total of twenty amino acids that your body needs. Most are nonessential, which means your body can make them for itself; however, there are nine that are considered essential or semi-essential since your body cannot readily make them. Most meat and dairy-based proteins are complete proteins. Things like beef, chicken, pork, eggs, milk, and cheese proteins are all largely complete proteins. Plant-based proteins are usually incomplete in that they do not contain all twenty amino acids. This is not to say that plant-based proteins are inferior, quite the opposite, but the thing to know is that you have to consume a wide variety of plant-based proteins in order to get all twenty amino acids that your body requires. Now on to fats.

Fats are typically found in foods like meat, cheese, eggs, and nuts. Sadly, they have been falsely labeled as "*bad*." As I mentioned earlier under carbohydrates, eating fat does not make you fat unless, again, you are eating far in excess of your daily calorie requirements. Fats are necessary for many critical bodily functions both at the cellular and systemic levels within your body. At the cellular level, for example, they control how substances pass across individual cell membranes, while at the systemic level, they help to make and maintain necessary compounds like hormones, which in turn control various metabolic functions within your body.

Here is another way to look at how erroneous the current thinking is when it comes to eating fat. If eating fat made you fat simply because the tissues are the same, then why wouldn't eating muscle, or meat, make you muscular in the same manner—without the need to work out?

Now I bet you are thinking to yourself, *"But, what about cholesterol?"* So as everyone pretty much knows, there are two key compounds related to cholesterol, HDL and LDL. HDL is an abbreviation for high-density lipoprotein, which is also known as *"good"* cholesterol. LDL is an abbreviation for low-density lipoprotein, or *"bad"* cholesterol. Both of these labels are misrepresentations of the function these two compounds perform within the body. Both HDL and LDL are necessary for many metabolic processes within the body. Here is a layman's explanation of how the two function. HDL travels around your body scavenging free cholesterol and returns it to your liver where it is reprocessed for distribution back out to where it is needed in your body. LDL is the vehicle that your body uses to deliver cholesterol from the liver to where it is needed throughout your body. So you can see, both are necessary, and neither is *"good"* or *"bad"*. The concept of good versus bad developed from the bonds that HDL and LDL use to carry cholesterol. The bonds in LDL are not as strong as the bonds in HDL, so occasionally cholesterol is released into your blood rather than at the location where it is required. But here is where HDL comes into play by scooping up and returning free cholesterol back to your liver for reprocessing.

Contrary to popular belief, cholesterol may not necessarily be the root cause of most heart disease all on its own. New science is now showing that erratic blood sugar levels have as much or more to do with heart disease than what was previously attributed to cholesterol alone.

It is now known that there is a direct link between heart disease and eating too many carbohydrates. Your body will convert excess carbohydrates into triglycerides so that they can be stored in fat cells. This in turn leads to an excess of both triglycerides and VLDL (very low-density lipoproteins) in your blood system. High levels of triglycerides are directly involved with the formation of plaque in your arteries. As I am sure you already know, this buildup of plaque in your arteries increases the risk of heart disease and stroke.

Now you see how carbohydrates are the hidden menace in nutrition planning. I know it sounds totally contrary to what you have been led to believe about nutrition, but it is true, and I have personally experienced how excess carbohydrates can derail your fat-burning plans regardless of how hard or long you work out.

Over the years I have tried many different diet and nutrition plans. All of them included carbohydrates of some type and at some level. These were considered necessary to a healthy nutrition plan. Recently, just last year as a matter of fact, I fell for what was considered the *extreme* in diet plans. I tried the keto diet, and it worked—to a point. What I came to see was that it was not keto and only eating fat, and by the way, it's not Atkins and only eating protein either. It's actually very simple. It's just *not* eating carbs! I quickly saw that it was not eating a bunch of fat that was making my body burn fat; it was that I was not eating lots and lots of simple, processed carbohydrates. In fact, the fewer carbohydrates you consume, the faster you will burn fat. You do not have to replace the carbohydrates with fat to get your body to burn fat; you just need to break the blood sugar spike and crash cycle that causes your body to believe it needs body fat as a storage device. It is literally like flipping a light switch.

In keto, flipping this fat-burning light switch is known as ketosis, which is a state of metabolism where your body is using fat instead of sugar or protein to produce energy. The belief is that if you eat lots of fats, your body will switch to ketosis, which will in turn also burn body fat. I believe this is a false assumption. Just because you are consuming high amounts of fat in your nutrition plan does not necessarily mean that your body is going to burn body fat to produce energy even though it is in a state of ketosis. Quite the contrary may actually be the case. You could be in ketosis simply because your body only has dietary fat to use to produce energy, and this is not the same as burning body fat. In fact, when it comes to ketosis, there are several supplements that you can take to produce ketones, which does not necessarily mean that your body is even in a state of ketosis. Again this does not necessarily mean that you are burning body fat just because you are in this induced state of ketosis.

Your body digests everything and breaks it down into smaller building blocks that it then uses to produce energy and build and repair tissue, among other functions and processes. Being in ketosis only means that your body is using fat to produce energy. If you are consuming large quantities of fat, then this makes sense; however, it does not automatically mean that your body will burn your body fat stores too, in order to maintain a state of ketosis. The two are related but not directly connected in a conjoined process of producing energy while also burning body fat.

The Atkins diet purports the same fat-burning effects, but rather than consuming large quantities of fats, you consume large quantities of proteins. Both miss the point that it is not about either of those two macronutrients but only about the remaining third macronutrient—simple, processed carbohydrates.

This now brings us full circle back to macronutrient management with an effective nutrition plan. In the Eat More, Do Less, Get Fit plan, you begin by establishing your total daily calorie requirement. I will show you a simple formula that you can use to determine the appropriate number of calories to consume in an average day. Now the term *"average"* is used because no two days are exactly the same. Some days may be more stressful or physically active, requiring more calories, while other days may present situations where you consume more calories than needed based on your daily activities. Therefore, your daily calorie requirement may vary from day to day, but as long as you are able to stay within a predesignated calorie intake range based on your specific condition and goals, you will achieve your desired results.

There are several calorie calculators out there online, but this is the one I prefer. It is based on your current weight and activity level. My recommendation would be to err on the low side and work up from there depending on how you feel at the level that you have selected. It is normal if you are trying to burn fat to transform your body to experience a little hunger, but it should not be *extreme*.

Number of calories per pound of body weight per day

Activity Level	Lose	Maintain	Gain
Sedentary	10–12	12–14	16–18
Moderate	12–14	14–16	18–20
Active	14–16	16–18	20–22

Here is a sample formula for someone who is active and trying to lose weight. The person's range would be between fourteen and sixteen calories per pound of bodyweight. With a current body weight of 150 pounds, the calculation would be as shown below.

150 x 14 = 2100

150 x 16 = 2400

The daily range would be between 2,100 and 2,400 calories to be allotted among the three macronutrient groups. The exact distribution would depend on your specific fitness goals and training program. We will discuss the macronutrient breakdown next.

There are many variants of calculating your target daily calorie requirements, but in the beginning, these general guidelines will work for almost everyone unless you have special dietary needs or concerns. As you progress, you may need to make modifications to these basic guidelines to better *"tune"* your nutrition plan to match your goals. This will make itself evident as you become more in tune with how your body feels and what it is telling you it needs. Yes. Your body will send you signals as to what it needs you to eat. The trick is to not confuse these signals with your cravings. Especially when it comes to simple, processed carbohydrate-rich foods.

The next step is to determine the appropriate number of calories per macronutrient. This is where it can become a bit of a challenge, but only in the very beginning. As I mentioned earlier, you need to train your body to understand that it does not need body fat as a storage device in order to deal with blood sugar spikes and crashes. If your goal is to burn body fat, in order to do this, you will need to control the number of simple, processed carbohydrates that you consume. In this case, less is best! For me, what I discovered was that if I set a target to eat zero carbs, and I know this now sounds *extreme*, I was able to significantly reduce but not totally eliminate carbohydrates. This enabled me to very quickly flip the fat-burning light switch to *"On"*, and I began to see almost immediate results. The reason being, the sooner you can flip the fat-burning light switch to *"On"*, the faster you will see results and the more your motivation will grow.

My reasoning was kind of like this: I saw it literally like a light switch in your home. It is either on or off—no in-betweens. Now this is not a permanent state where you will never be able to eat carbohydrates like cake, cookies, ice cream, pasta, or bread again. It is just a short-duration retraining period for your body so that it realizes that it does not need body fat. Once the fat-burning light switch has been flipped to *"On"*, you can go back and eat foods like these again. The trick is to *not* eat simple, processed carbohydrates on a regular basis and flip the fat-burning light switch back to *"Off"*.

If you go back to eating simple, high-glycemic carbohydrates on a regular basis, you will retrain your body to make and retain fat because the repetitive spikes and crashes will recreate the old norm where your body once again believes it needs body fat. If you can switch away from simple, processed carbs to more protein, fat, and complex, high-fiber, low-glycemic-index carbohydrates on a regular basis, you can stray every now and then and enjoy your favorite simple carbohydrates without flipping the fat-burning light switch back to *"Off"*. The key is to only do this intermittently and on an irregular basis so your body will not recognize any sort of pattern. Occasional simple, processed carbohydrate consumption will not tell your body to start making and retaining fat as long as you do not do it repetitively several times a day every day. What I do is save these types of foods for special occasions and celebrations, and believe me, there are plenty of those in life that you will not miss out on these types of foods.

This is where Eat More, Do Less, Get Fit diverges from almost all other health and fitness programs.

In contrast, most programs believe in a high level of carbohydrates coupled with long and arduous cardio sessions to burn fat. Eat More, Do Less, Get Fit utilizes a more effective balanced macronutrient nutrition plan coupled with an efficient training routine so that you can truly *Eat More, Do Less, Get Fit*!

Determining the best macronutrient split is specific to each individual. For me, I have found that if I simply try to avoid carbohydrates altogether, I end up eating enough since they are found in most food sources anyway. The key thing to remember here is that your goal is to reduce your *"net carbohydrate"* intake. To determine net carbohydrates, you simply subtract the number of grams of fiber from the total number of carbohydrates in the food you are eating. The result is the net carbohydrates contained in that food source.

To draw a comparison, according to the keto diet, you should consume no more than forty net carbohydrates in a single day. The belief is that eating any more than forty net carbohydrates will kick you out of ketosis, and the fat-burning process will cease. Here again, I believe ketosis is not the actual fat-burning process that your body uses to eliminate body fat. It is the reduction in carbohydrates that flips the fat-burning light switch to the *"On"* position that burns body fat. So limiting yourself to only forty net carbohydrates is not really necessary with Eat More, Do Less, Get Fit. It is much more a personal choice and journey for each person.

An initial macronutrient split could be something like this, but again this is only a starting point and may need to be adjusted on an individual basis.

Protein   40–50%

Fats   40–50%

Carbohydrates   10–20% (Remember, less is best here.)

In addition to macronutrients, food also consists of micronutrients, phytonutrients, and zoonutrients (if you eat meat). Each of these also plays an important role in nutrition planning. Let's begin with micronutrients.

Micronutrients are compounds like vitamins and minerals that are required in far smaller quantities but are essential as catalysts for most bodily processes, including metabolism. They work hand in hand with macronutrients throughout the body.

Phytonutrients are additional compounds that are found only in plants. These natural substances include carotenoids such as lutein, flavonoids, isoflavones, and plant sterols, to name a few. These natural compounds provide antioxidants and improve both your immune system and hormonal function.

Zoonutrients are natural molecules found in dairy and animal food sources. They have been shown to play a key role in several critical body processes, including anti-inflammatory, antihypertension, and antimicrobial actions, as well as contributing to the quality of your digestion and immune systems. Both CoQ10 and collagen are prime examples of zoonutrients.

Nutrition planning not only includes food but also hydration. Hydration is critical to a sound nutrition plan. I am sure you have heard that you need to drink 120 ounces of water each day. This sounds like a lot, but in actuality it is not. Consider that water is in almost every beverage that you drink. For instance, if you use protein powder supplements, then you are probably mixing them with water, so that counts toward your daily total. If you consider all the sources of water that you drink in the day other than just water, you will see that it is much easier than assumed at first glance to drink about 120 ounces of water a day. I have found that drinking a glass or bottle of water first thing in the morning is very beneficial because you have just gone several hours without a single drink while you were sleeping.

As a side note to hydration, there is another reason why limiting the amount of carbohydrates you consume in a day is beneficial. In order for your body to process one gram of carbohydrate, your body requires two grams of water! Yes. That is a lot of water that you will need to consume in order to just process the carbohydrates that you eat. And that's not all. Just imagine how bloated you will be if you are eating a large number of carbohydrates on a regular basis. So much for a lean physique, right?

Another area where a lot of misinformation exists concerns alcohol and whether or not it is good for you. This all depends on your health and fitness goals along with your desire to achieve them. Alcohol can significantly impact your health and fitness efforts when it comes to your nutrition planning and how it affects your body's metabolic processes.

Calories from alcohol are known as *"empty"* calories because they do not contain any nutrients like amino acids, vitamins, or minerals, and when compared to macronutrients, they are also somewhat high in calories. If you recall, proteins and carbohydrates have four calories per gram, and fat has nine. Alcohol has seven calories per gram, and when combined with its little to no nutritional value, alcohol is really not beneficial to your nutrition plan.

There is another aspect of alcohol consumption that compounds its effects on metabolism—especially fat-burning. Alcohol is quickly absorbed by the body. Approximately 20 percent is almost immediately absorbed through tissues in the mouth and stomach, subsequently reaching the brain in about a minute! The remaining 80 percent has to be metabolized by your liver, which will metabolize alcohol before macronutrients since it is considered a toxin by the body. Alcohol is metabolized from acetaldehyde into acetate to be excreted by the body, and this prioritization slows the fat-burning process because the liver is now metabolizing alcohol instead of fat since it cannot store the calories for later use like it can with macronutrients. Even worse, science has shown that alcohol specifically decreases fat-burning around your belly, giving credence to the term *"beer belly"*!

Because the liver is now processing alcohol, blood sugar levels will also drop since macronutrients are no longer being processed into glucose (energy) for the body. Additionally, your body can only process about one ounce of liquor per hour. If you are consuming at a higher rate, alcohol will build up in the blood and other body tissues, including your brain, until it can be metabolized. This will prolong alcohol's interference with both healthy metabolism and fat-burning.

Now I am not saying you can never have another adult beverage, but drinking on a regular basis, just like eating simple, processed, high-glycemic carbohydrates on a frequent basis, will certainly have a negative impact on your nutrition planning and overall health and fitness goals. Save alcohol, like cake and ice cream, for celebrating special occasions. As with processed carbohydrates, there are plenty of special occasions to keep you satisfied, trust me.

You now see how important nutrition planning is and how much it will impact your ability to reach your desired fitness goals. Nutrition planning will create the conditions within your body to burn excess body fat to reveal the muscular development you have achieved through your physical training. I will not kid you; this process does initially require some degree of personal discipline when it comes to avoiding simple, processed carbohydrates, but once you get the fat-burning light switch to flip to the *"On"* position, you will see immediate results, which will motivate you to continue until you reach your personal fitness goals. Later on in the chapter on Living the Eat More, Do Less, Get Fit Life, I will give you some simple tips and tricks that I personally employed to enable me to be disciplined and flip the fat-burning light switch to *"On"*. By following the Eat More, Do Less, Get Fit nutrition plan, you can do it too. *Eat More*!

CHAPTER 2:
TRAINING

When it comes to training, there are several factors that come into play. First and foremost, you have to define what your objectives are so that you can set corresponding goals and then apply the appropriate training methodology. For instance, I believe that most people say they want to *"get in shape,"* but what they really mean is that they want to *"reshape"* their bodies while also improving their cardiovascular performance. However, this is usually not well communicated and translates into a perceived desire to follow pop culture workouts as if they were training for a CrossFit competition or Spartan Race with *extreme* training regimens. There is little middle-of-the-road training, and most fitness enthusiasts believe in *extreme* hardcore training. This is simply not necessary for the average person trying to achieve modest gains in appearance and health. Actually, almost quite the opposite is a more effective and efficient method of training.

It is important to identify what sort of result you truly want. For instance, there is nothing wrong with wanting to train for a CrossFit competition; however, that sort of training is significantly different than training for, say, a power-lifting competition or a bikini contest. I see four distinct types of training: cardio/endurance, athletic performance, powerlifting and bodybuilding, and then body-shaping. Each has its own method of training that will enable you to reach your personal goals. I am going to focus on the body-shaping style of training, as I believe that is more closely aligned with most people's goals.

Along with an appropriate training methodology, rest and recovery are just as important as the actual physical training itself. Physical training places stress on your body, and in order to heal, your body will need days to recuperate and rebuild, regardless of your specific training methodology.

Now, rest and recovery days do not necessarily mean lie around all day in front of the TV. It simply means that on these days you should not do any physical training that significantly works any muscle tissue that is already stressed. Your body will utilize the calories that you consume on these days to heal itself and rebuild your fast-twitch muscle as you work to reshape it. Your body is made of two types of muscle fiber, slow-twitch and fast-twitch. We will discuss the two types of muscle fiber and how they relate to different training methodologies a little later on in this chapter.

On your *"off"* days, you can do things like stretch, go for a walk, practice yoga, or do balance training poses—just as long as you do not strain yourself. This is the *Do Less* part of the program. The secret here is to keep moving, but not at a workout level or pace. This will maintain your body's fluidity and prevent you from stiffening up. It will also be a great way to relieve any muscle pain that you might have incurred from your progressive weight-training workouts.

Another aspect of rest is getting a full night's sleep. Your body requires a minimum eight hours of sleep per night in order to recover from your training program. Training actually damages muscle tissue, and your body repairs itself while you sleep. This is the muscle soreness that you feel on the next day and how your body builds fast-twitch muscle. By stressing your muscle tissue, the cells are forced to both grow in size and multiply, thus shaping your physique. So if you are not getting enough sleep, your body is not afforded the opportunity to fully heal itself, which will detract from your physical training and impair your ability to achieve your fitness goals.

Unlike cardio training that works your slow-twitch muscle fiber, progressive weight training works your fast-twitch muscle tissue, which is where you will need to focus if you are trying to reshape your body. Fast-twitch muscle is the lean tissue that your body uses for short bursts of energy, like in lifting weights and sprinting, where your body applies maximum effort for a very short period of time. Fast-twitch muscle tissue, unlike slow-twitch, can be built and shaped via a process called *"hypertrophy"* which is just a fancy term for muscle building. Please do not confuse muscle building with bodybuilding type physiques. Although the two methods of training are similar and both utilize progressive weight training, bodybuilding is by far and away a much more *extreme* version of training than body-shaping. That is why I grouped it with powerlifting.

As I mentioned earlier, physical training does not have to be *extreme* to work. I prefer progressive weight training as the best means to accomplish body reshaping. To that end, here is what I would propose as a starting point for beginners. More experienced individuals who already have an established training routine may find some of this helpful or may choose to follow their current routine. Nothing in Eat More, Do Less, Get Fit is mandatory.

I would recommend a staggered workout schedule along with what is known as the *PUSH-PULL-LEGS* program. This is a program that organizes the muscles that you will train during each workout based on the idea that you will be training muscles that are complementary to each other in the same workout. This is the breakdown:

PUSH is exactly what it sounds like. These are all the muscles in your upper body that you use to push things away from yourself: chest, shoulders, and triceps.

PULL is the opposite. These are all the muscles that you would use to pull something toward yourself: upper back and biceps.

LEGS is just that. On this day you train just your lower body with a range of exercises that will work your entire leg: front of your thighs, back of your thighs, butt, and calves.

For a beginner, the best schedule to follow initially is a three-day-per-week training schedule. For instance, you could train on Monday, Wednesday, and Friday or Tuesday, Thursday, and Saturday. These are the very popular schedules in that it also gives you a day of rest in between each workout and then two days of total rest on the weekend to fully recover before the next week's workouts. This alternating-days schedule is a large part of the *Do Less* concept. First off, you do not need to be in the gym for hours on end. My recommendation would be no more than thirty minutes per workout to start. As you progress and begin to reshape your body, you may notice areas that you might want to focus on with a few more extra sets, so your workouts could extend to forty-five minutes, but I would say that no more than an hour is about the max time for a workout. That is only one and a half to three hours of training per week.

For some people, as they progress through their body reshaping journey, their goals may change, and they may consider moving into what I would consider the bodybuilding or powerlifting modes of training. These require more than just three workouts per week and are part of a perfectly natural transition, but they are not something we are going to cover since that is not necessarily geared for the average Joe.

Now, if you would like to add some cardio to your routine, that is perfectly fine, but remember to stay within your target fat-burning heart rate zone. Cardio-style training does not train the same lean tissue as progressive weight training. Cardio trains what is known as slow-twitch muscle fiber. Slow-twitch muscle fiber is used by the body to perform repetitive low-power movements like walking, running, etc. and will not *"shape"* your body. Slow-twitch muscle tissue is not prone to grow in size, but rather becomes more efficient at producing and utilizing energy to prolong the repetitive motion it is intended to provide.

I would also recommend doing this cardio separately from your weight training so as to not detract from your body-shaping workout by burning the energy that your body will need for power during the progressive weight training sessions. The best time to incorporate cardio is first thing in the morning—before breakfast. I know this is beginning to sound *extreme*, but it is actually very simple and not that demanding. There are several benefits to doing your cardio first thing in the morning. In this way it will not detract from your weight training sessions, which are best for body reshaping goals but will kick-start your metabolism first thing in the morning so that you will metabolically burn more calories throughout the day.

My recommendation for this early morning cardio training is short and sweet. Just do about fifteen to twenty minutes of some sort of exercise.

Depending on what is available to you, you can do a short elliptical or treadmill session, you can do a high-repetition ab workout, or you can simply go for what is known as a "*fasted walk*", which is just a quick-paced walk before eating your first meal of the day. Remember—this does not have to be extreme in any way but rather works best if you maintain your target fat-burning heart rate zone. Here, too, this early morning cardio does not need to be performed in the gym. Identifying exercises that you can do at home to accomplish this workout is best to minimize the total time required for these cardio workout sessions.

An added benefit is that by splitting your cardio from your weight training in this manner, you will shorten the time you need to be in the gym during any given workout. Instead of spending one to one and a half hours in the gym all at once, you only need to be there for maybe thirty to forty minutes. In addition, since we all live hectic lives and things do pop up that could interfere with your training schedule, by utilizing two smaller workouts in a day, you will always work out at least for fifteen to twenty minutes on your workout days. This fail-safe will help to keep your body from falling into the "*use lean tissue*" mode to fuel itself.

Lastly, I would like to dispel a popular myth about cardio training and fat-burning when it comes to the belief that you can follow a poor nutrition plan and compensate by doing more intense and longer cardio workouts. This is simply not the case and at best simply creates a calorie deficit that can be better accomplished through nutrition planning. If you consume too many simple, processed carbohydrates in your nutrition plan, your body will still experience blood sugar spikes and crashes, which send messages to your body that it needs body fat. No matter what sort of cardio workout you pursue, it will not send the signal to your body to burn body fat. Your body will simply send you back signals to consume more carbohydrate-rich foods or, worse yet, utilize lean tissue to compensate for the increased calorie requirements. Besides, why create a scenario with poor nutrition where you have to spend even more time in the gym trying to burn those excess carbohydrate-related calories?

I personally no longer do any repetitive cardio, like elliptical, treadmill, or running—at all. The closest I come to cardio is my ab training, which for me is intended to provide core stability for other exercises like squats, shoulder presses, etc. rather than cardio.

I know this sounds like a big commitment, and at first it may seem that way, but it is a worthwhile commitment that you are making to yourself that will provide huge benefits in every area of your life. These recommendations are only a starting point and nothing is mandatory. Maybe two workout sessions in one day is too much, or maybe you prefer to do all of your training at the same time. The beauty here is that the physical training aspect of Eat More, Do Less, Get Fit is that you do not have to work out like a professional bodybuilder. The secret is to just be regular about it. Try not to miss two days in a row except during your initial schedule where weekends are designated for rest and recovery if you are on the Monday-Wednesday-Friday workout schedule.

The three-days-per-week routine that I have presented is a good starting point. Many people will feel this is enough for them as they accomplish their personal fitness goals. Others may decide to strive for new fitness goals based on their accomplishments. If you become the latter, there are many, many training routines and modifications that can be made to the nutrition plan to enable you to go as far as you want.

Now I know a lot of women are now saying or thinking, *"But I don't want to get big and bulky like those bodybuilders."* I understand this concern, but now I would also like to put it to rest. Women's bodies do not produce testosterone the same way men's bodies do, and therefore, you are not really able to get big and muscular like a man. You can, however, build muscle in a more limited fashion, which is exactly what you want to do if you are trying to reshape your body into a lean physique. Progressive weight training will not necessarily make you big and bulky, unless you decide to train to do so and also take supplements to encourage your body to produce more testosterone than normal.

I have seen many women in the gym trying to trim down by endless hours of cardio training on treadmills, ellipticals, or bikes but neglecting to train their upper bodies in any meaningful way. Sadly, this is the exact opposite of what needs to be done to affect the change that they are seeking. To trim your body below the waist and create more of a V-shape versus the archetypal female pear-shape physique, the best method is to train both your upper and lower body. If you only train your lower body in an attempt to trim down, your upper body will atrophy. "*Atrophy*" is a technical term for "*wither away*". Your body will actually consume this lean upper body tissue because it will interpret the lack of training of this muscle as a lack of necessity to carry it on your body. This will in turn only accentuate the pear-shaped physique that most women are trying so hard to reshape through long and arduous cardio sessions.

The amazing thing about progressive weight training is that it actually occurs within your fat-burning target heart rate zone. This makes progressive weight training ideal for burning body fat and makes doing cardio unnecessary for body reshaping. The first step in benefiting from working out within your fat-burning target heart rate zone is to determine your fat-burning target heart rate zone.

In order to determine your fat-burning target heart rate zone, you will first need to begin with determining your resting heart rate. To do this, sit with your legs uncrossed and feet flat on the floor. Take a couple smooth breaths and try to relax. Find your pulse and count the number of beats for fifteen seconds and then multiply this number by four to determine your resting heart rate. Repeat this process three times to get a good average of you resting heart rate. Now use that number in the formula below to calculate your max heart rate and fat-burning target heart rate zone.

Max heart rate calculation:

[(220–your age)–your resting heart rate] + (1 + your resting heart rate)

Target fat-burning heart rate zone:

75% to 85% of your max heart rate

Sample calculation:

Age: 58

Resting heart rate: 72

[(220–58)–72] * (1 + 72) = (162-72) + 73 = 163

Minimum fat-burning heart rate:

75% of max = 163 * 0.75 = 122

Maximum fat-burning heart rate:

85% of max = 163 * 85% = 139

Target fat-burning heart rate zone = 122–139

    The most effective fat-burning heart rate range for the example above is 122–139, but for simplicity's sake you can round to 125–140. This is the range that the person from this example would want to stay within when performing their cardio workouts. If you do not have a heart rate monitor or are not using equipment that does, a good way to estimate this range is that when you are training, you should be able to carry on a conversation with little to moderate effort in conjunction with the increased labored breathing caused by the demands of your workout.

    Now for more of the *Do Less* part of Eat More, Do Less, Get Fit. When you are performing your progressive weight training routines, your heart rate will most likely enter this same target heart rate range. Yes. Progressive weight training utilizes short bursts of energy at near maximum effort, but you also rest in between sets. Even though this training elevates your heart rate, it usually does not raise it above your target heart rate zone, and if it does, it is only momentarily, and your heart rate quickly returns to the appropriate range. Sort of like a mini-HIIT (high intensity interval training) cycle. Furthermore, since progressive weight training is based on sets and reps, you can easily manage your workout to maintain your target heart rate zone.

Another aspect of training that you will hear about quite often is *"core training"*. To me, this means *"balance training"*, as opposed to ab training. Many trainers will have you doing multiple concurrent movements to *"engage"* your core. I am skeptical of this at best in that it seems to only complicate the base movement and detract from the results. I would encourage you to use balance movements such as yoga, but if yoga is not your thing, then there are lots of alternative activities and exercises that you can do to build your balance.

Balance is not an innate thing that you lose as you get older. What actually happens is the small muscles that your body uses to maintain its balance start to atrophy due to lack of use. When you were younger you probably participated in sports in school or just played outside in the backyard. Or maybe you just danced a lot more when you were younger. As we get older and work takes over a large percentage of our time, we find ourselves sitting far more than we are designed to do. This is how these *"balance"* muscles atrophy. You just need to start using them again, and to be honest, it does not require a lot of effort. Just a few minutes a couple times per week, on your rest days for example, play some pick-up basketball or badminton to casually add some agility training into your life. There are even several simple exercises or poses that you can do that are specifically designed to improve balance. A simple online search for *"balance poses"* or *"balance exercises"* will produce endless results. Any of these activities will work to adequately build your balance without the need to combine weightlifting moves with risky unsteady stances.

So as you have just seen, the training part of Eat More, Do Less, Get Fit is really quite simple and not all that demanding. The time requirement can range anywhere from a couple hours per week to as many as you like, with the average falling somewhere around five to six hours per week, split between quick morning cardio workouts and evening progressive weight training across three different days.

Also, if you goal is to burn fat and reshape your body, as is most people's, then once you have burned the fat away, you can modify your workout program to either maintain what you have accomplished or push yourself further to see what you can do now that you know how. Reaching this point is a huge accomplishment that you should and will be very proud of achieving. Where you go from there is totally up to you. *Do Less*!

CHAPTER 3:
MY STORY

I am sure, as I often am when I read someone else's manifesto on an important topic, that you are curious about my story. Well, here it is.

I will start way back when I was in high school. As I mentioned earlier, I was the quintessential ninety-pound weakling. I decided at that time to pursue bodybuilding and powerlifting, which I did for several years. I even competed in the very first Mr. Grand Rapids (Michigan) bodybuilding competition at the Green Apple Bar. Those of you from Grand Rapids will understand just how long ago that was.

I continued to lift weights and eat everything in sight in my attempt to weigh 200 pounds. I will tell you that I was successful in my quest and actually achieved a body weight of 210 pounds. That occurred while I was in college around the age of twenty-five. After college I joined the Army, where running became the epitome of physical training. As you can well guess, weighing 210 pounds while trying to run miles and miles was a direct contradiction. So I began to lean out and dropped down to about 175 pounds. While I was in the Army, I got married, and this started the inevitable yo-yoing of body weight and on-again, off-again working out.

For the next several years, I flipped back and forth between working out and not working out—mostly not working out. But more importantly, I also fell into a horrible nutrition pattern where I did not monitor anything that I ate. This lasted through my thirties and early forties. Then, in my early forties, I decided that because I was now divorced, I needed to maintain some sort of physical appeal to women, so I began to train much more seriously. I also began to look at different diets at this time. This is where I first encountered the frustration of starving myself and still not eliminating body fat the way I wanted. Over the course of my forties and then into my fifties, I continued to combine weightlifting along with significant cardio in the hopes of trimming down my body fat. Not only was I unsuccessful, but I also incurred several repetitive-motion, cardio-training related injuries that culminated in serious damage to my IT bands after running a half marathon.

For those of you who know what IT bands are, you will understand the seriousness of this issue. If you do not, here is a quick explanation. Your IT bands (iliotibial bands) run the length of your outer thigh and significantly influence the movement of your hip along with stabilizing your knees. I bring this up now because this injury led me to a point where I was no longer able to work any muscles below the waist, and I did not want to be one of those guys in the gym with a big chest and arms but chicken legs. So, in a state of depression, I decided to quit training altogether since I was also now in my mid-fifties. I figured, what's the point, you know?

This decision impacted me in several ways—most of them not good. It did, however, allow my IT bands to heal, somewhat, but the negative emotional and psychological impacts were far greater. I had several personal and professional issues going on at this same time, so many so, that my friend Jason once said, ,*"you need a magazine rack to hold them all"*, and together, they all led me into a life-changing decision. It was at this point that I decided to get back into shape as a means of grounding myself. To me, working out is very much like meditation because it forces you to focus on the exercise movement and exclude everything else from your mind. This is also when I decided to pursue the keto diet, which triggered my realization that simple, processed carbohydrates were the real culprits behind body fat. Once I realized this fact, it then became my personal mission to bring this to as many people as I could, and thus the impetus for this book.

I quickly realized while on the keto diet that it was not about eating large amounts of fat but rather eating fewer carbohydrates in order to avoid blood sugar spikes and crashes. Along with this realization, I also saw that working out did not have to be nearly as intense or time consuming as popular opinion purported. Instead, I quickly realized that cardio was not necessary and that progressive weight training on a much more relaxed schedule would work just as well for me to accomplish my goals.

Now if you ask any of my friends and family, they will tell you that I am a very decisive and determined person, and that proved to be a huge benefit in my journey. Once I decide to do something, nothing will stand in my way. I am also a very regimented person, which helped when it came to my nutrition planning and physical training. I am very accustomed to routine and monotony. Now this in no way means your journey has to be monotonous; in fact, I chose monotony because I am somewhat lazy when it comes to food preparation. I prefer simple and easy to do, which translates into eating the same thing over and over. I do not recommend this as a course of action unless it is how you approach things in general already. Trust me when I say there are plenty of foods out there to choose from so that you do not become bored with your nutrition plan.

For me, I basically chose to eat eggs and bacon for breakfast and then meat and salads for the other meals in the day. I would regularly swap out salads for vegetables like broccoli, asparagus, or my newfound favorite, brussels sprouts. My Mom will laugh when she reads that because when I was young, we would throw brussels sprouts at each other across the dinner table. I had four brothers, so I am sure you can see it happening! I was very repetitive in my food selection for my nutrition plan, but that does not mean that you have to be too.

For snacks during the day, I relied upon almonds, cocktail peanuts, and Cheese Whisps. Another favorite snack of mine is Duke's Smoked Shorty Sausages. All of these snacks are high in either protein, fat, or both. I also supplemented my meals with casein protein powder drinks.

By sticking to very few carbs the majority of the time, I am able to also enjoy what I call *"cheat carbs"* during the week on an occasional basis. I will go out and have fajitas with all the tortilla chips or swing by a local favorite restaurant of mine called BJs for a Pizookie. For those of you that do not know, a Pizookie is a freshly baked cookie with a scoop of ice cream on top, and there are several varieties to choose from so you never get bored. *Yum!* Cheddar's restaurants have a similar cookie dessert, and it is just as delicious! Can you tell I have a horrible sweet tooth the size of Montana? That is pretty much it for my nutrition plan, simple and straightforward. The physical training that I do is pretty much this simple too.

At first, when it came to working out, I trained twice per day—yes, way too *extreme*. I was still caught up in the old way of thinking about working out and calorie deficits as they relate to burning body fat. I did a fifteen- to twenty-minute cardio workout that consisted of three five-minute HIIT elliptical sets or a twenty- to thirty-minute bike ride every day before work in the early morning and then progressive weight training in the evening five days per week. My after-work evening weight-lifting routine was a three days-on, one day-off Push-Pull-Legs routine. After several weeks of this *"two-a-day"* routine, I realized this was not necessary. In fact, this *extreme* activity, in particular the cardio, actually began to irritate my IT bands again. So I discontinued any sort of cardio workout that required repetitive leg movements like running, riding, or elliptical. Instead, I began to work my abs as a form of early-morning cardio. I also reduced the number of early-morning workouts to just two or three per week depending on my three on, one off schedule.

This is currently how I train with the exception of how I stagger the days. I now follow a six-days-on, one-day-off schedule and train each body part twice per week. My cardio ab workouts are still only two to three days per week. I am training a little heavier now than what is necessary to shape my body because I have decided to gain some muscle. Again, this is not necessary but rather a personal choice that I have made.

On a final note, I earned my ISSA Personal Trainer and Nutrition Specialist certifications as part of my journey to educate myself further about fitness and nutrition. This was more a personal goal and by no means a requirement for you to be successful in your personal fitness journey. In fact, I have just related a large part of what I learned from my certification training to you in this book.

Now that you know my story, go out and create your own health and fitness success story!

Eat More, Do Less, Get Fit!

CHAPTER 4:
LIVING THE EAT MORE, DO LESS, GET FIT LIFESTYLE

So now I'm sure you are thinking things like "*Okay, you have made some great points—now how do I put it all together?*" or "*Surely you don't expect me to not eat carbs ever again for the rest of my life?*" Putting it all together to live the life that you envision is actually quite easy. You now know much more about nutrition and how to work out. Now it is all up to you to live the Eat More, Do Less, Get Fit life that is right for you. You get to decide what is right for you and how you want to go about accomplishing your health and fitness goals.

The important factor in all of this is that you are in control. Each person that reads this book and applies these techniques will experience their own individual journey. You get to be in charge. Not the diet, not your personal trainer, not your body—but *you*! This subtle change in your life will not only enable you to accomplish your personal fitness goals, but also give you the confidence to take control of other areas of your life where you might feel a need for change.

Remember, training is the easy part, and nutrition is the foundation. Going forward, more attention will need to be applied to your continued nutrition planning than perhaps your physical training, unless you decide that once you have achieved your initial goals, you set the bar a little higher and want to further define your physique. But even in this scenario, nutrition will still be the key, and training will simply evolve into the routine that will enable you to accomplish your new fitness goals. Whether it be continued body-shaping, cardio endurance, athletic performance, or strength training, all of these are reliant upon your nutrition planning.

Now, about carbohydrates. In no way are you prohibited from eating carbohydrates. As I stated very early on, other than the initial few weeks that are necessary to flip the fat-burning light switch to *"On"*, you can eat carbohydrates as you see fit. The only caveat here is that you must eat them intelligently. Be sure to only eat low glycemic index carbohydrates like oatmeal, apples, and bananas. Do not eat them regularly throughout the day so that you avoid creating a pattern of blood sugar spikes and crashes that your body will interpret as a need to make and retain body fat. Once you successfully flip the fat-burning light switch to *"On"*, then your body will begin to crave proteins and fats rather than simple, processed carbohydrates. That is why I recommended saving dessert-type carbohydrates for special occasions—not every meal.

This sounds much more difficult than it truly is. You will quickly see there are lots and lots of special occasions that involve what I call *"cheat carbs"*. I personally found myself, and I never thought this would ever happen, actually craving salads on a regular, almost daily basis. I would catch myself saying things like *"I have not had a salad yet today"* while at the same time feeling a strong *"need"* for a very large salad.

As long as you are diligent and do not reestablish the pattern of eating carbohydrates where your body falls back into believing it needs body fat to compensate, then you are good to go. It is really that simple. You can proverbially *"have your cake and eat it too!"*

As I proceeded through my Eat More, Do Less, Get Fit journey, I discovered a couple of very simple tips and tricks that helped me through some of those tough times when I was trying to get the fat-burning switch to flip to the *"On"* position.

One thing that helped me was that I was able to discover alternative foods like cocoa dusted almonds to help get over the inevitable *"I need a dessert"* hump. That small nagging craving to satisfy your sweet tooth, if you have one. This was my greatest challenge. I have the worst sweet tooth!

I found cocoa-dusted almonds to be just the trick to get me over the hump. Lots of protein and fat with minimal carbs, but still able to satisfy my sweet-tooth craving.

Another trick I used was to go out and eat the foods that I have craved for so long but was convinced would *"make me fat"* due to their high fat content. Once I realized this was not the case, I was able to enjoy foods like fried chicken wings, ribeye steaks, brats, cheese, eggs, sausage of all kinds, and of course *bacon*! I began to eat bacon as often as I could. It was almost like cheating since the current prevailing thought is that eating fat will make you fat!

There is also a side benefit to all of this too. When friends, acquaintances, coworkers, and family begin to see you burning body fat and getting into shape, they will undoubtedly ask about your *"diet"*. The look that you will see on everyone's face will be truly entertaining when you begin to describe your nutrition plan. And this leads me back to another point that is critical to your success.

When you start your journey, you will be surrounded by everyone you now know. Some will truly be supportive, others will be supportive but in a negative way, and then there will be those that will outright try to discourage you from your journey. The best advice I can give to help counter any negativity you encounter is to first find a partner who is interested in achieving similar results. This has many benefits. Not only will having a partner help you with everything from emotional and spiritual support to training and maintaining your nutrition plan, but this will also give you the opportunity to help them to do the same. I have found that this is the very best method to enable you to follow your health and fitness path as well as counter the naysayers that you will inevitably encounter along the way. It is like teaching and learning. The best way to learn is to teach.

Now a word about naysayers. Naysayers come in a couple different forms. From coworkers and even family members who will dispute what you now know to be the truth to those who will call you crazy for wanting to eat healthy and avoid eating things like donuts and soda. This is all a defense mechanism for them to avoid accepting the fact that they do not possess the same inner strength that you are now displaying on your journey.

This will cause them to feel a sense of disappointment with themselves, for which they will subsequently hold you responsible so that they can feel justified in focusing their discomfort toward you. This will emerge as an attempt to dissuade you from working to accomplish your goals in order to make themselves feel better about their lack of inner strength to do the same. Remember, this says way more about them than it does about you.

My suggestion would be to seek out like-minded people who are on the same sort of health and fitness journey that you are pursuing. There are several online websites and groups that provide wonderful support and advice. Seek them out because they will help keep you motivated and also provide continued health and fitness education.

Once you begin your health and fitness journey, I am sure you will want to track your progress more than just by looking at yourself in the mirror. Most people will want to monitor their weight in order to track their progress. I am here to tell you this is probably not the best way to "*see*" what you have accomplished because as you begin to burn body fat and add muscle, you will actually get thinner, but may also get heavier. Yes. This is true. Body fat is much less dense than muscle tissue. That means body fat takes up much more "*space*" on your body than muscle.

I can best illustrate this by comparing a cubic foot of feathers with a cubic foot of lead. The feathers represent body fat while the lead represents lean muscle. A cubic foot of feathers weighs only a few pounds, depending on the specie of bird, while a cubic foot of lead weighs 708 pounds! The same "*space*" but with considerably different weights. That is why it is more representative to gauge your progress with measurements and clothes sizes rather than weight. I personally prefer clothes measurements since all I have to do is put on my current clothes and watch as they become way too big! Maybe the one downside to getting into shape is that you have to continuously buy new clothes throughout your health and fitness journey.

Now you have it all. It is up to you to start the journey. Good luck and have fun!

Eat More, Do Less, Get Fit!

CHAPTER 5:
SUPPLEMENTS

There are a multitude of supplements that you can take that will assist in many aspects of your health and fitness journey. They will not only ensure a complete nutrition plan but also provide compounds that can improve your training and recovery. They range from protein powders to vitamins to other compounds scientifically proven to have beneficial effects when coupled with a sound nutrition plan and physical training. Here is a list of just a few that I believe are worth considering as part of your health and fitness program.

BCAAS (BRANCH CHAIN AMINO ACIDS)
These supplements consist of only three essential amino acids: Leucine, Isoleucine, and Valine. These three amino acids are basic building blocks of lean tissue.

CREATINE
This is a natural substance that increases muscle mass, boosts strength, and enhances exercise performance.

EAAS (ESSENTIAL AMINO ACIDS)
These consist of all nine essential amino acids: Lysine, Methionine, Phenylalanine, Threonine, Tryptophan, Leucine, Isoleucine, Valine, and Histidine. Recent science has shown that your body actually needs all nine amino acids to produce lean tissue.

PRE-WORKOUT
There are several good pre-workout supplements on the market that contain various ingredients such as vitamins, minerals, BCAAs, CLA, Creatine, Beta-alanine, etc. These are designed to enhance your workout in order to maximize results.

POST-WORKOUT
Similar to pre-workout supplements, there are several of these on the market that aid in post-workout recovery.

PROTEIN POWDERS
Whey: protein derived from milk that is quickly absorbed by the body. Best used before a workout or right afterward.

Casein: another milk-based protein that is more slowly absorbed by the body. Because of this, it is best taken before bed so that your body will have a source of protein as it rebuilds itself during the night.

Vegan: protein supplements derived from plants that are equal to animal-based proteins as long as you get a full amino-acid supplement that contains all twenty amino acids.

MICRONUTRIENTS

VITAMINS
Multivitamins: to ensure that all vitamins, even trace vitamins, are consumed.

B Vitamins: used by the body in energy production.

Vitamin C: used to repair tissue and as an anti-inflammatory.

Vitamin D: necessary for bone health, immune system function, and regulating insulin levels.

Vitamin E: believed to be an antiaging nutrient utilized by the immune system and as an anti-inflammatory.

MINERALS
Magnesium: important for many processes in the body, including regulating muscle and nerve function, blood sugar levels, and blood pressure, along with making protein, bone, and DNA.

Potassium: one of the most important minerals in the body. It helps regulate fluid balance, muscle contractions, and nerve signals.

Zinc: helps the immune system and plays a role in cell division, cell growth, and wound healing.

OTHER COMPOUNDS
Glucosamine: a natural compound that helps maintain and repair cartilage.

Hyaluronic Acid: found in your skin, connective tissue, and eyes, where its main function is to retain moisture to keep tissues lubricated, which improves mobility.

CLA (Conjugated Linoleic Acid): a compound used to help reduce fat, build muscle, and increase both energy and endurance.

NADS (Nicotinamide Adenine Dinucleotide): an antiaging supplement.

Turmeric: a natural substance that helps reduce inflammation.

Probiotics: digestive supplement that not only improves digestion but also aids in other body processes, such as the immune system.

Holy Basil and Ashwagandha: two herbal supplements that help relieve stress.

www.ingramcontent.com/pod-product-compliance
Lightning Source LLC
LaVergne TN
LVHW011900060526
838200LV00054B/4450